The complete Lean and green diet cookbook

Delicious dessert and salad recipes that anyone can make

Lisa Reims

Table of contents

DESSERT AND SALAD 7

Chocolate Bars 7

Blueberry Muffins 9

Chia Pudding.. 11

Avocado Pudding 12

Delicious Brownie Bites... 14

Wasabi Tuna Asian Salad 17

Lemon Greek Salad.. 19

Broccoli Salad 21

Potato Carrot Salad.. 23

Marinated Veggie Salad... 26

Mediterranean Salad 29

Potato Tuna Salad.. 31

High Protein Salad... 33

Rice and Veggie Bowl... 35

Squash Black Bean Bowl.. 38

Pea Salad.. 42

Snap Pea Salad... 45

Cucumber Tomato Chopped Salad.. 47

Zucchini Pasta Salad.. 49

Egg Avocado Salad 51

Sweet Potato Muffins Fueling Hack 52

Asian Cabbage Salad 55

Tangy Kale Salad 57

Crunchy Cauliflower Salad... 59

Crisp Summer Cucumber Salad....................................... 61

Decadently Dark Chocolate Mousse 63

Fresh Strawberry Salad Dressing.................................... 65

Pumpkin Balls 66

Smooth Peanut Butter Cream 68

Vanilla Avocado Popsicles.. 70

Chocolate Popsicle 72

Raspberry Ice Cream... 74

Chocolate Almond Butter Brownie 76

Peanut Butter Fudge 78

Almond Butter Fudge.. 81

Homemade Coconut Ice Cream 82

Coconut Panna Cotta... 85

Blueberry Lemon Cake.. 87

Rich Chocolate Mousse 90

Raspberry Cheesecake... 92

Peanut Butter Brownie Ice Cream Sandwiches......................95

Chocolate Frosty 97

Tiramisu Milkshake 99

Weight Watchers Macaroni Salad Recipe with Tuna...........100

Big Mac Salad...103

Loaded Caesar Salad with Crunchy Chickpeas 105

Shrimp Cobb Salad 107

Fruit Salad..109

Strawberry, Orange & Rocket Salad 110

Strawberry & Asparagus Salad 113

DESSERT AND SALAD

Chocolate Bars

Prep Time: 10 minutes

Cook Time: 20 minutes

Serve: 16

Ingredients:

- 15 oz cream cheese, softened
- 15 oz unsweetened dark chocolate
- 1 tsp vanilla
- 10 drops liquid stevia

Instructions:

1.Grease 8-inch square dish and set aside.

2.In a saucepan, dissolve chocolate over low heat.

3.Add stevia and vanilla and stir well.

4.Remove pan from heat and set aside.

5.Add cream cheese into the blender and blend until smooth.

6.Add melted chocolate mixture into the cream cheese and blend until just combined.

7.Transfer mixture into the prepared dish and spread evenly, and place in the refrigerator until firm.

Nutrition: Calories: 230 Fat: 24 g Carbs: 7.5 g Sugar: 0.1 g Protein: 6 g Cholesterol: 29 mg

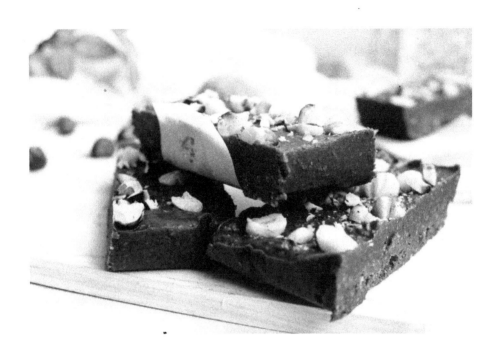

Blueberry Muffins

Prep Time: 15 minutes

Cook Time: 35 minutes

Serve: 12

Ingredients:

- 2 eggs
- 1/2 cup fresh blueberries
- 1 cup heavy cream
- 2 cups almond flour
- 1/4 tsp lemon zest
- 1/2 tsp lemon extract
- 1 tsp baking powder
- 5 drops stevia
- 1/4 cup butter, melted

Instructions:

1.heat the cooker to 350 F. Line muffin tin with cupcake liners and set aside.

2.Add eggs into the bowl and whisk until mix.

3.Add remaining ingredients and mix to combine.

4.Pour mixture into the prepared muffin tin and bake for 25 minutes.

Nutrition: Calories: 190 Fat: 17 g Carbs: 5 g Sugar: 1 g Protein: 5 g Cholesterol: 55 mg

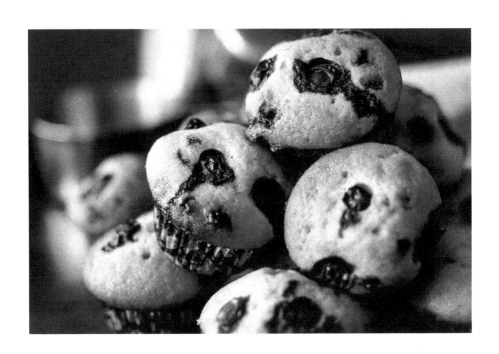

Chia Pudding

Prep Time: 20 minutes

Cook Time: 0 minutes

Serve: 2

Ingredients:

- 4 tbsp chia seeds
- 1 cup unsweetened coconut milk
- 1/2 cup raspberries

Instructions:

1. Add raspberry and coconut milk into a blender and blend until smooth.

2. Pour mixture into the glass jar.

3. Add chia seeds in a jar and stir well.

4. Seal the jar with a lid and shake well and place in the refrigerator for 3 hours.

5. Serve chilled and enjoy.

Nutrition: Calories: 360 Fat: 33 g Carbs: 13 g Sugar: 5 g Protein: 6 g Cholesterol: 0 mg

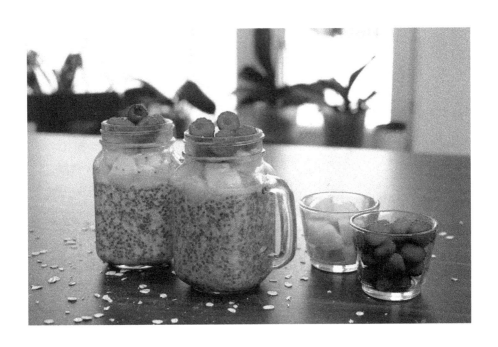

Avocado Pudding

Prep Time: 20 minutes

Cook Time: 0 minutes

Serve: 8

Ingredients:

- 2 ripe avocados, pitted and cut into pieces
- 1 tbsp fresh lime juice
- 14 oz can coconut milk
- 2 tsp liquid stevia
- 2 tsp vanilla

Instructions:

1.Inside the blender, Add all ingredients and blend until smooth.

Nutrition: Calories: 317 Fat: 30 g Carbs: 9 g Sugar: 0.5 g Protein: 3 g Cholesterol: 0 mg

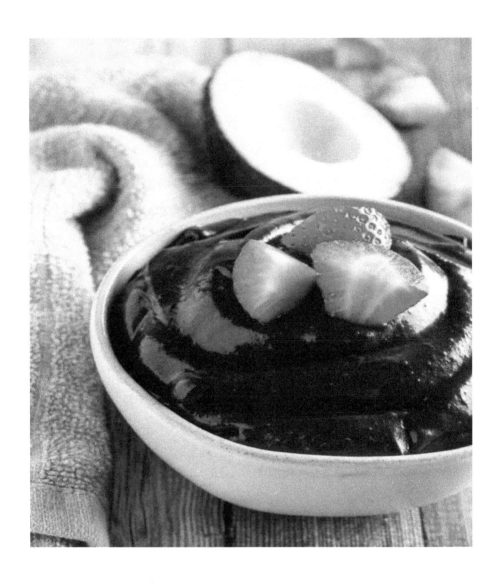

Delicious Brownie Bites

Prep Time: 20 minutes

Cook Time: 0 minutes

Serve: 13

Ingredients:

- 1/4 cup unsweetened chocolate chips
- 1/4 cup unsweetened cocoa powder
- 1 cup pecans, chopped
- 1/2 cup almond butter
- 1/2 tsp vanilla
- 1/4 cup monk fruit sweetener
- 1/8 tsp pink salt

Instructions:

1.Add pecans, sweetener, vanilla, almond butter, cocoa powder, and salt into the food processor and process until well combined.

2.Transfer the brownie mixture into the large bowl. Add chocolate chips and fold well.

3.Make small round shape balls from brownie mixture and place them onto a baking tray.

4.Place in the freezer for 20 minutes.

Nutrition: Calories: 108 Fat: 9 g Carbs: 4 g Sugar: 1 g Protein: 2 g Cholesterol: 0 mg

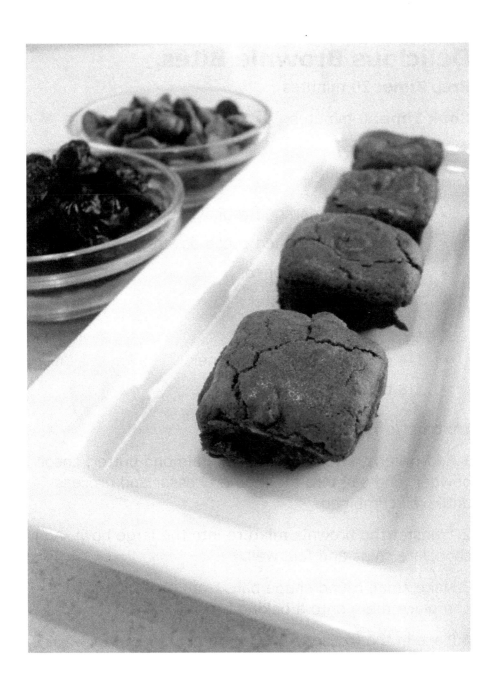

Wasabi Tuna Asian Salad

Prep Time: 30 minutes

Cook Time: 10 minutes

Serve: 1

Ingredients:

- Lime juice (1 teaspoon)
- Non-stick cooking spray
- Pepper/dash of salt
- Wasabi paste (1 teaspoon)
- Olive oil (2 teaspoons)
- Chopped or shredded cucumbers (1/2 cup)
- Bok Choy stalks (1 cup)
- Raw tuna steak (8 oz.)

Instructions:

1.Fish: preheat your skillet to medium heat. Mix your wasabi and lime juice; coat the tuna steaks.

2.Use a non-stick cooking spray on your skillet for 10 seconds.

3.Put your tuna steaks on the skillet and cook over medium heat until you get the desired doneness.

4.Salad: Slice the cucumber into match-stick tiny sizes. Cut the bok Choy into minute pieces. Toss gently with pepper, salt, and olive oil if you want.

Nutrition: Protein: 61g, Fiber: 1g, Cholesterol: 115mg, Saturated fats: 2g, Calories: 380

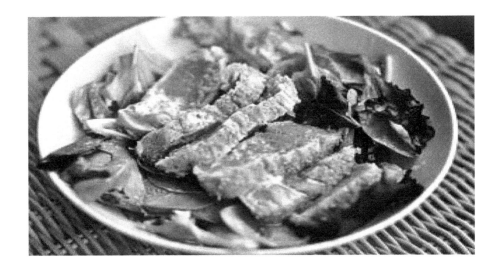

Lemon Greek Salad

Prep Time: 25 minutes

Cook Time: 25 minutes

Serve: 1

Ingredients:

- Chicken breast (140 oz)
- Chopped cucumber (1 cup)
- Chopped orange/red bell pepper (1 cup)
- Wedged/sliced/chopped tomatoes (1 cup)
- Chopped olives (1/4 cup)
- Fresh parsley (2 tablespoons), finely chopped.
- Finely chopped red onion (2 tablespoons)
- Lemon juice (5 teaspoons)
- Olive oil (1 teaspoon)
- Minced garlic (1 clove)

Instructions:

1.Preheat your grill to medium heat.

2.Grill the chicken and cook on each side until it is no longer pink or for 5 minutes.

3.Cut the chicken into tiny pieces. In your serving bowl, mix garlic, olives, and parsley. Whisk in olive oil (1 teaspoon) and lemon juice (4 teaspoons). Add onion, tomatoes, bell pepper, and cucumber.

4.Toss gently. Coat the ingredients with dressing. Add another teaspoon of lemon juice to taste. Divide the salad into two servings and put 6oz chicken on top of each salad.

Nutrition: Protein: 56g, Fiber: 4g, Total carbs: 14g, Sodium: 280mg, Cholesterol: 145mg, Saturated fat: 2.5g, Total fat: 12g, Calories: 380

Broccoli Salad

Prep Time: 5 minutes

Cook Time: 25 minutes

Serve: 1

Ingredients:

- 1/3 tablespoons sherry vinegar
- 1/24 cup olive oil
- 1/3 teaspoons fresh thyme, chopped
- 1/6 teaspoon Dijon mustard
- 1/6 teaspoon honey
- Salt to taste
- 1 1/3 cups broccoli florets
- 1/3 red onions
- 1/12 cup parmesan cheese shaved
- 1/24 cup pecans

Instructions:

1.Mix the sherry vinegar, olive oil, thyme, mustard, honey, and salt in a bowl.

2.In a serving bowl, blend the broccoli florets and onions.

3.Drizzle the dressing on top.

4.Sprinkle with the pecans and parmesan cheese before serving.

Nutrition: Calories: 199, Fat: 17.4g, Saturated fat: 2.9g, Carbohydrates: 7.5g, Fiber: 2.8g, Protein: 5.2g

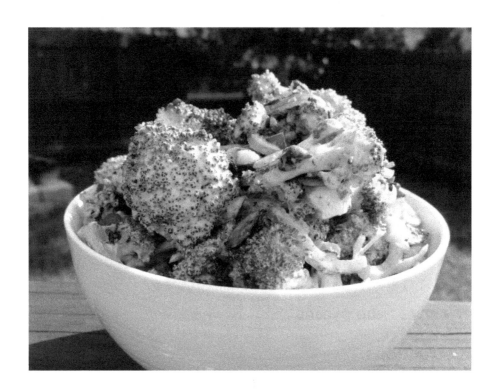

Potato Carrot Salad

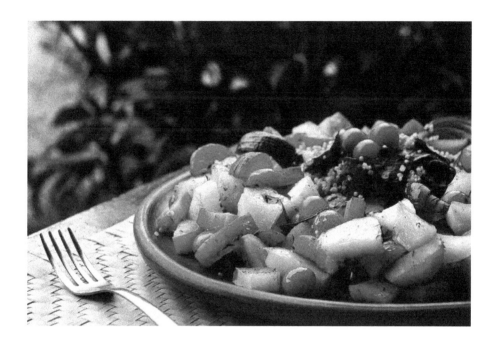

Prep Time: 15 minutes

Cook Time: 10 minutes

Serve: 1

Ingredients:

Water

- 1 potato, sliced into cubes
- 1/2 carrots, cut into cubes

- 1/6 tablespoon milk
- 1/6 tablespoon Dijon mustard
- 1/24 cup mayonnaise

Pepper to taste

- 1/3 teaspoons fresh thyme, chopped
- 1/6 stalk celery, chopped
- 1/6 scallions, chopped
- 1/6 slice turkey bacon, cooked crispy and crumbled

Instructions:

1.Fill your pot with water.

2.Place it over medium-high heat.

3.Boil the potatoes and carrots for 10 to 12 minutes or until tender.

4.Drain and let cool.

5.In a bowl, mix the milk, mustard, mayonnaise, pepper, and thyme.

6.Stir in the potatoes, carrots, and celery.

7.Coat evenly with the sauce.

8.Cover and refrigerate for 4 hours.

9.Top with the scallions and turkey bacon bits before serving.

Nutrition: Calories: 106, Fat: 5.3g, Saturated fat: 1g, Carbohydrates: 12.6g, Fiber: 1.8g, Protein: 2g

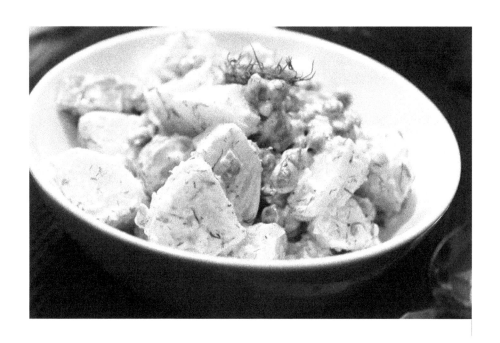

Marinated Veggie Salad

Prep Time: 4 hours and 30 minutes

Cook Time: 3 minutes

Serve: 1

Ingredients:

- 1 zucchini, sliced
- 4 tomatoes, sliced into wedges
- ¼ cup red onion, sliced thinly
- 1 green bell pepper, sliced
- 2 tablespoons fresh parsley, chopped
- 2 tablespoons red-wine vinegar
- 2 tablespoons olive oil
- 1 clove garlic, minced
- 1 teaspoon dried basil
- 2 tablespoons water
- Pine nuts, toasted and chopped

Instructions:

1.In a bowl, combine the zucchini, tomatoes, red onion, green bell pepper, and parsley.

2.Pour the vinegar and oil into a glass jar with a lid.

3.Add the garlic, basil, and water.

4.Seal the jar and stir well to combine.

5.Pour the dressing into the vegetable mixture.

6.Cover the bowl.

7.Marinate in the refrigerator for 4 hours.

8.Garnish with the pine nuts before serving.

Nutrition: Calories: 65, Fat: 4.7g, Saturated fat: 0.7g, Carbohydrates: 5.3g, Fiber: 1.2g, Protein: 0.9g

Mediterranean Salad

Prep Time: 20 minutes

Cook Time: 5 minutes

Serve: 1

Ingredients:

- 1 teaspoon balsamic vinegar
- 1/2 tablespoon basil pesto
- 1/2 cup lettuce
- 1/8 cup broccoli florets, chopped
- 1/8 cup zucchini, chopped
- 1/8 cup tomato, chopped
- 1/8 cup yellow bell pepper, chopped
- 1/2 tablespoons feta cheese, crumbled

Instructions:

1.Arrange the lettuce on a serving platter.

2.Top with the broccoli, zucchini, tomato, and bell pepper.

3.In a bowl, mix the vinegar and pesto.

4.Drizzle the dressing on top.

5.Sprinkle the feta cheese.

Nutrition: Calories: 100, Fat: 6g, Saturated fat: 1g, Carbohydrates: 7g, Protein: 4g

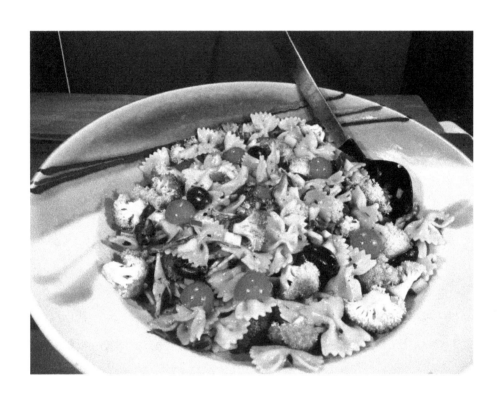

Potato Tuna Salad

Prep Time: 4 hours and 20 minutes

Cook Time: 10 minutes

Serve: 1

Ingredients:

- 1 potato, peeled and sliced into cubes
- 1/12 cup plain yogurt
- 1/12 cup mayonnaise
- 1/6 clove garlic, crushed and minced
- 1/6 tablespoon almond milk
- 1/6 tablespoon fresh dill, chopped
- ½ teaspoon lemon zest
- Salt to taste
- 1 cup cucumber, chopped
- ¼ cup scallions, chopped
- ¼ cup radishes, chopped
- (9 oz) canned tuna flakes
- 1/2 hard-boiled eggs, chopped
- 1 cups lettuce, chopped

Instructions:

1. Fill your pot with water.

2. Add the potatoes and boil.

3. Cook for 15 minutes or till slightly tender.

4.Drain and let cool.

5.In a bowl, mix the yogurt, mayo, garlic, almond milk, fresh dill, lemon zest, and salt.

6.Stir in the potatoes, tuna flakes, and eggs.

7.Mix well.

8.Chill in the refrigerator for 4 hours.

9.Stir in the shredded lettuce before serving.

Nutrition: Calories: 243, Fat: 9.9g, Saturated fat: 2g, Carbohydrates: 22.2g, Fiber: 4.6g, Protein: 17.5g

High Protein Salad

Prep Time: 5 minutes

Cook Time: 5 minutes

Serve: 1

Ingredients:

Salad:

- 1(15 oz) can green kidney beans
- 1/4 tablespoon capers
- 1/4 handfuls arugula
- 1(15 oz) can lentils

Dressing:

- 1/1 tablespoon caper brine
- 1/1 tablespoon tamari
- 1/1 tablespoon balsamic vinegar
- 2/2 tablespoon peanut butter
- 2/2 tablespoon hot sauce
- 2/1 tablespoon tahini

Instructions:

For the dressing:

1.In a bowl, stir all the ingredients until they come together to form a smooth dressing.

For the salad:

2.Mix the beans, arugula, capers, and lentils. Top with the dressing and serve.

Nutrition: Calories: 205, Fat: 2g, Protein: 13g, Carbs: 31g, Fiber: 17g

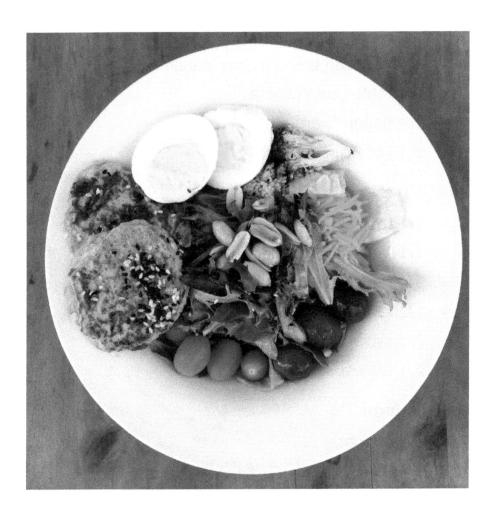

Rice and Veggie Bowl

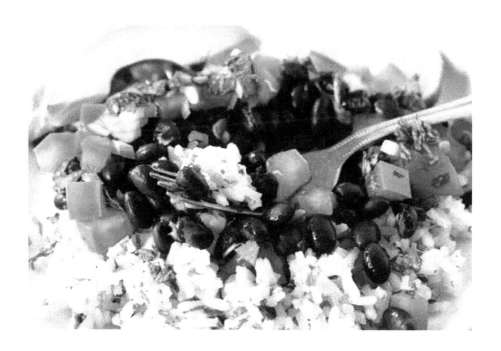

Prep Time: 5 minutes

Cook Time: 15 minutes

Serve: 1

Ingredients:

- 1/3 tablespoon coconut oil
- 1/2 teaspoon ground cumin
- 1/2 teaspoon ground turmeric
- 1/3 teaspoon chili powder
- 1 red bell pepper, chopped

- 1/2 tablespoon tomato paste
- 1 bunch of broccoli, cut into bite-sized-florets with short stems 1/2 teaspoon salt, to taste
- 1 large red onion, sliced
- 1/2 garlic cloves, minced
- 1/2 head of cauliflower, sliced into bite-sized florets 1/2 cups cooked rice
- Newly ground black pepper to taste

Instructions:

1.Start with warming up the coconut oil over medium-high heat.

2.Stir in the turmeric, cumin, chili powder, salt, and tomato paste.

3.Cook the content for 1 minute. Stir repeatedly until the spices are fragrant.

4.Add the garlic and onion. Fry for 2,5 to 3,3 minutes until the onions are softened.

5.Add the broccoli, cauliflower, and bell pepper. Cover, then cook for 3 to 4 minutes and stir occasionally.

6.Add the cooked rice. Stir so it will combine well with the vegetables. Cook for 2 to 3 minutes. Stir until the rice is warm.

7.Check the seasoning and change to taste if desired.

8.Lessen the heat and cook on low for 2 to 3 more minutes so the flavors will meld.

9.Serve with freshly ground black pepper.

Nutrition: Calories: 260, Fat: 9g, Protein: 9g, Carbs: 36g, Fiber: 5g

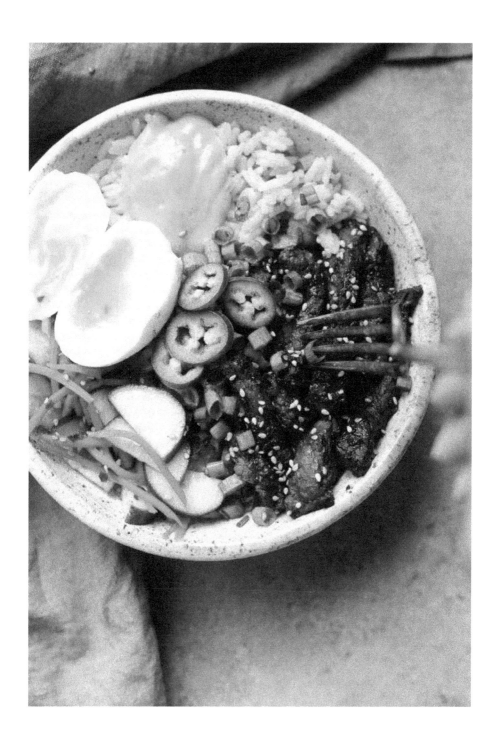

Squash Black Bean Bowl

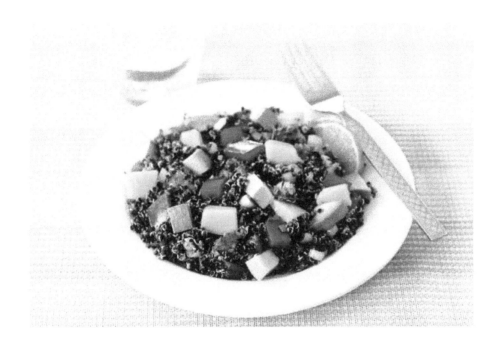

Prep Time: 5 minutes

Cook Time: 30 minutes

Serve: 1

Ingredients:

- 1 large spaghetti squash, halved,
- 1/3 cup water (or 2 tablespoon olive oil, rubbed on the inside of squash)

Black bean filling:

- 1/2 (15 oz) can of black beans, emptied and rinsed

  1/2 cup fire-roasted corn (or frozen sweet corn)

  1/2 cup thinly sliced red cabbage
- 1/2 tablespoon chopped green onion, green and white parts ¼ cup chopped fresh coriander
- ½ lime, juiced or to taste
- Pepper and salt, to taste

Avocado mash:

- One ripe avocado, mashed
- ½ lime, juiced or to taste
- ¼ teaspoon cumin
- Pepper and pinch of sea salt

Instructions:

1.Preheat the oven to 400°F.

2.Chop the squash in part and scoop out the seeds with a spoon, like a pumpkin.

3.Fill the roasting pan with 1/3 cup of water. Lay the squash, cut side down, in the pan. Bake for 30 minutes until soft and tender.

4.While this is baking, mix all the ingredients for the black bean filling in a medium-sized bowl.

5.In a small dish, crush the avocado and blend in the avocado mash ingredients.

6. Eliminate the squash from the oven and let it cool for 5 minutes. Scrape the squash with a fork so that it looks like spaghetti noodles. Then, fill it with black bean filling and top with avocado mash.

Nutrition: Calories: 85, Fat: 0.5g, Protein: 4g, Carbs: 6g, Fiber: 4g

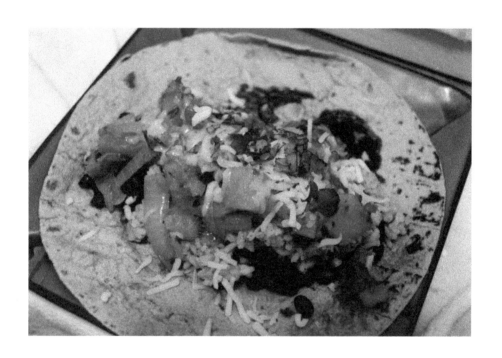

Pea Salad

Prep Time: 40 minutes

Cook Time: 0 minutes

Serve: 1

Ingredients:

- 1/2 cup chickpeas, rinsed and drained
- 1/2 cups peas, divided
- Salt to taste
- 1 tablespoon olive oil
- ½ cup buttermilk
- Pepper to taste
- 2 cups pea greens
- 1/2 carrots shaved
- 1/4 cup snow peas, trimmed

Instructions:

1. Add the chickpeas and half of the peas to your food processor.

2. Season with salt.

3. Pulse until smooth. Set aside.

4. In a bowl, toss the remaining peas in oil, milk, salt, and pepper.

5. Transfer the mixture to your food processor.

6. Process until pureed.

7.Transfer this mixture to a bowl.

8.Arrange the pea greens on a serving plate.

9.Top with the shaved carrots and snow peas.

10.Stir in the pea and milk dressing.

11.Serve with the reserved chickpea hummus.

Nutrition: Calories: 214, Fat: 8.6g, Saturated fat: 1.5g, Carbohydrates: 27.3g, Fiber: 8.4g, Protein: 8g

Snap Pea Salad

Prep Time: 1 hour

Cook Time: 0 minutes

Serve: 1

Ingredients:

- 1/2 tablespoons mayonnaise
- ¾ teaspoon celery seed
- ¼ cup cider vinegar
- 1/2 teaspoon yellow mustard
- 1/2 tablespoon sugar
- Salt and pepper to taste
- 1 oz. radishes, sliced thinly
- 2 oz. sugar snap peas, sliced thinly

Instructions:

1.In a bowl, combine the mayonnaise, celery seeds, vinegar, mustard, sugar, salt, and pepper.

2.Stir in the radishes and snap peas.

3.Refrigerate for 30 minutes.

Nutrition: Calories: 69, Fat: 3.7g, Saturated fat: 0.6g, Carbohydrates: 7.1g, Fiber: 1.8g, Protein: 2g

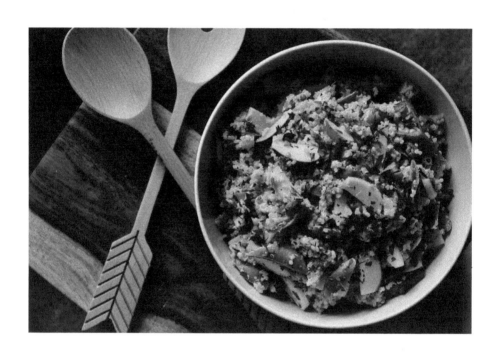

Cucumber Tomato Chopped Salad

Prep Time: 15 minutes

Cook Time: 0 minutes

Serve: 1

Ingredients:

- 1/4 cup light mayonnaise
- 1/2 tablespoon lemon juice
- 1/2 tablespoon fresh dill, chopped
- 1/2 tablespoon chive, chopped
- 1/4 cup feta cheese, crumbled
- Salt and pepper to taste
- 1/2 red onion, chopped
- 1/2 cucumber, diced
- 1/2 radish, diced
- 1 tomato, diced
- Chives, chopped

Instructions:

1.Combine the mayonnaise, lemon juice, fresh dill, chives, feta cheese, salt, and pepper in a bowl.

2.Mix well.

3.Stir in the onion, cucumber, radish, and tomatoes.

4.Coat evenly.

5.Garnish with the chopped chives.

Nutrition: Calories: 187, Fat: 16.7g, Saturated fat: 4.1g, Carbohydrates: 6.7g, Fiber: 2g, Protein: 3.3g

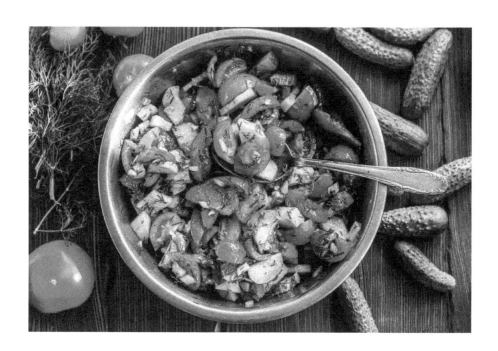

Zucchini Pasta Salad

Prep Time: 4 minutes

Cook Time: 0 minutes

Serve: 1

Ingredients:

- 1 tablespoon olive oil
- 1/2 teaspoons dijon mustard
- 1/3 tablespoons red-wine vinegar
- 1/2 clove garlic, grated
- 2 tablespoons fresh oregano, chopped
- 1/2 shallot, chopped
- ¼ teaspoon red pepper flakes
- 4 oz. zucchini noodles
- ¼ cup Kalamata olives pitted
- 1 cups cherry tomato, sliced in half
- ¾ cup parmesan cheese shaved

Instructions:

1.Mix the olive oil, Dijon mustard, red wine vinegar, garlic, oregano, shallot, and red pepper flakes in a bowl.

2.Stir in the zucchini noodles.

3.Sprinkle on top the olives, tomatoes, and parmesan cheese.

Nutrition: Calories: 299, Fat: 24.7g, Saturated fat: 5.1g, Carbohydrates: 11.6g, Fiber: 2.8g, Protein: 7g

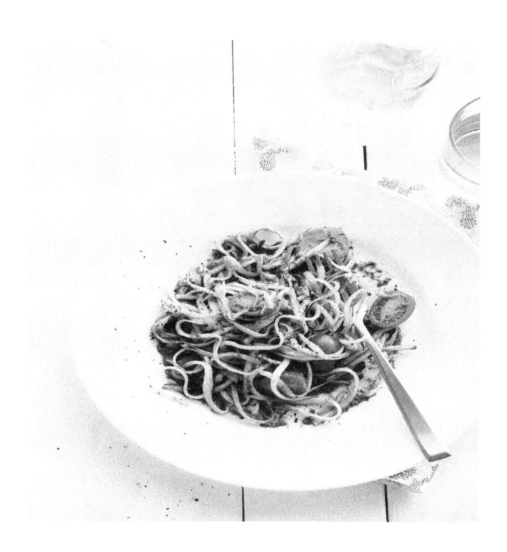

Egg Avocado Salad

Prep Time: 10 minutes

Cook Time: 0 minutes

Serve: 1

Ingredients:

- 1/2 avocado
- 1 hard-boiled egg, peeled and chopped
- 1/4 tablespoon mayonnaise
- 1/4 tablespoons freshly squeezed lemon juice ¼ cup celery, chopped
- 1/2 tablespoons chives, chopped
- Salt and pepper to taste

Instructions:

1. Add the avocado to a large bowl.

2. Mash the avocado using a fork.

3. Stir in the egg and mash the eggs.

4. Add the mayonnaise, lemon juice, celery, chives, salt, and pepper.

5. Chill in the refrigerator for at least 2o to 30 minutes before serving.

Nutrition: Calories: 224, Fat: 18g, Saturated fat: 3.9g, Carbohydrates: 6.1g, Fiber: 3.6g, Protein: 10.6g

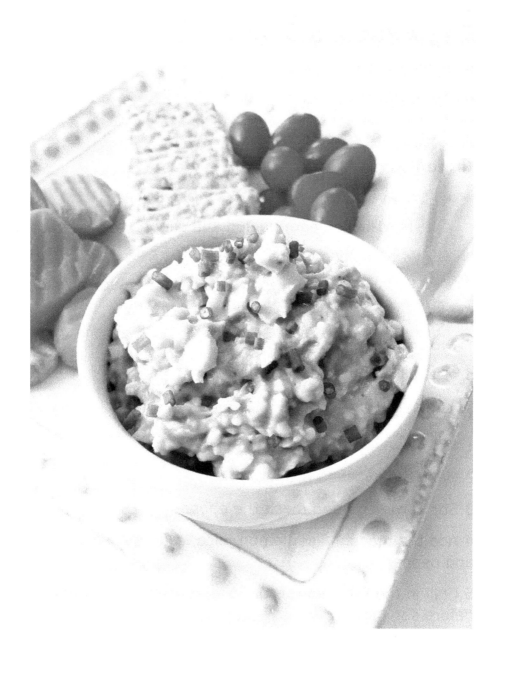

Sweet Potato Muffins Fueling Hack

Prep Time: 15 minutes

Cook Time: 15 minutes

Serve: 4

Ingredients:

- 1 packet Honey Sweet potatoes
- 2 Tablespoon liquid egg (like Eggbeaters) 1/2 C water
- 1/4 tsp baking powder
- 2 pinches Sinful Cinnamon Seasoning

Instructions:

1. Preheat oven to 400 degrees.

2. Sift the baking powder into the liquid egg.

3. Puree the sweet potatoes and add to the egg/baking powder mix.

4. Go on a light run and bring the water to a boil; add to the potato mix.

5. Bring in the cinnamon and the seasoning.

6. Whisk until well-combined.

7. Fill about ¾ of the way with the muffin cups with this mix.

8. Place into the oven for 15 minutes.

Nutrition: Energy (calories): 189 kcal Protein: 39.52 g Fat: 10.02 g Carbohydrates: 1.98 g Calcium, Ca44 mg Magnesium, Mg48 mg Phosphorus, P200 mg

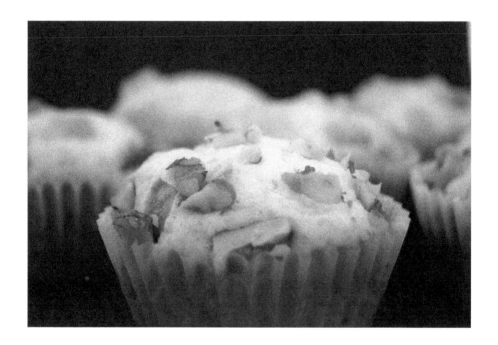

Asian Cabbage Salad

Prep Time: 10-15 minutes

Cook Time: 2 minutes

Serve: 4-8

Ingredients:

- 4 C green-cabbage, shredded
- 1/4 C rice wine-vinegar (no sugar added) 1 Tablespoon low sodium soy-sauce
- 4 little spoon Stacey Hawkins Valencia Orange Oil (optional- can be made fat free simply by leaving out)
- 1 normal spoon Asian style seasoning 2 teaspoons lime juice
- 1/4 C cilantro, chopped to taste with salt and pepper

Instructions:

1.Combine shredded cabbage with shredded cabbage in a large bowl, green onions, cilantro, citrus dressing, and Asian seasoning (seeds removed, ground In a coffee grinder, or in a pestle and mortar, with a pestle); mix well. Chill in the refrigerator.

Nutrition: Energy (calories): 99 kcal Protein: 4.13 g Fat: 4.53 g Carbohydrates: 12.47 g Calcium, Ca92 mg Magnesium, Mg35 mg Phosphorus, P95 mg

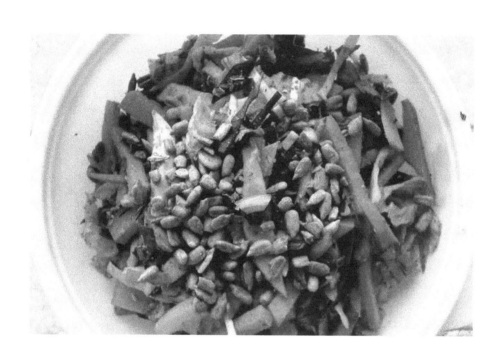

Tangy Kale Salad

Prep Time: 20 minutes

Cook Time: 6 minutes

Serve: 6

Ingredients:

- One-half cup olive oil
- One-fourth cup lemon juice 2 tablespoons Dijon mustard 1 tablespoon minced shallot
- 1 small garlic clove, finely minced
- One-fourth teaspoon salt, or more to taste ground black pepper to taste

Salad:

- 1 teaspoon olive oil
- One-third cup sliced almonds
- 1 bunch kale, center stems discarded and leaves thinly sliced 8 ounces Brussels sprouts, shredded
- 1 cup grated Pecorino Romano cheese

Instructions:

1.Whisk together the lemon Juice to create the dressing, olive oil, shallot, garlic, mustard, ¼ teaspoon salt and pepper. Set aside.

2.To make the salad, heat the oil over medium-high heat in a large skillet. Add the almonds and cook, sometimes stirring, until the almonds are cooked.

Almonds are ready. They are fragrant, and the oil is very aromatic about 2 minutes. Transfer to a plate. Attach the skillet to the kale and cook until it begins to wilt and become colorful for about 4 minutes.

3.Add the Brussels sprouts, reduce the heat to medium-low. Season with salt and pepper. Stuff the leaves with the cheese. Drizzle with the dressing.

4.Top with the almonds.

Nutrition: Energy (calories): 193 kcal Protein: 1.74 g Fat: 19.11 g Carbohydrates: 5.56 g Calcium, Ca23 mg Magnesium, Mg14 mg

Crunchy Cauliflower Salad

Prep Time: 10 minutes

Cook Time: 10 minutes

Serve: 8

Ingredients:

- 4 cups cauliflower florets
- 1 Tablespoon (one capful) Stacey Hawkins Tuscan Fantasy Seasoning
- 1/4 cup apple cider vinegar

Instructions:

In a wide bowl,

1.Position the cauliflower florets and coat them with a vinegar solution. Add Stacey Hawkins Tuscan Fantasy Seasoning and stir well. Let sit to allow cauliflower to marinate for 10 minutes.

2.Preheat the oven to 450 degrees and Put a baking sheet on top of it—heavy-duty foil. On a baking sheet, put the marinated cauliflower and bake in the 450-degree oven for 10-12 minutes. Remove and allow to cool.

Nutrition: Energy (calories): 29 kcal Protein: 1.72 g Fat: 0.24 g Carbohydrates: 5.36 g Calcium, Ca20 mg Magnesium, Mg13 mg Phosphorus, P39 mg

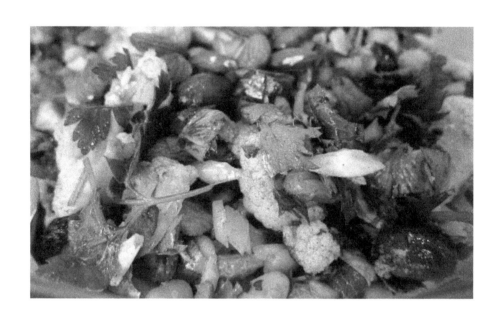

Crisp Summer Cucumber Salad

Prep Time: 15 minutes

Cook Time: 0 minutes

Serve: 4

Ingredients:

- 4 C sliced cucumbers (peels on or off- your choice)
  2 T apple cider vinegar
- 1/4 C sliced white onion
- 2 tsp Stacey Hawkins Dash of Desperation Seasoning

Instructions:

1.Reserve some cucumber slices for garnish.

2.In a tub, mix up the rest of the ingredients.

3.Pour over remaining cucumber slices and place in a pretty bowl.

4.Enable 15 minutes to sit down to absorb the flavor and serve.

Nutrition: Energy (calories): 20 kcal Protein: 0.29 g Fat: 0.53 g Carbohydrates: 3.08 g Calcium, Ca3 mg Magnesium, Mg3 mg Phosphorus, P6 mg

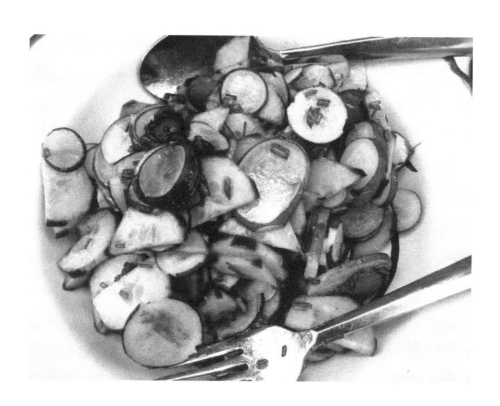

Decadently Dark Chocolate Mousse

Prep Time: 10 minutes

Cook Time: 0 minutes

Serve: 2

Ingredients:

- 2 ripe avocados
- One-half cup unsweetened, dark cocoa powder 1 T vanilla
- One-fourth cup stevia powder
- One-fourth cup Unsweetened pinch of almond milk salt

Instructions:

1.Combine all ingredients into a high-speed blender and blend until smooth. (This can be done in a food processor as well. I would skip the blending and just mash the ingredients with a mortar and pestle.)

2.Preserve this mousse in a closed container in the fridge for up to 5 days.

Nutrition: Energy (calories): 466 kcal Protein: 9.27 g Fat: 38.35 g Carbohydrates: 31.21 g Calcium, Ca132 mg Magnesium, Mg154 mg Phosphorus, P259 mg

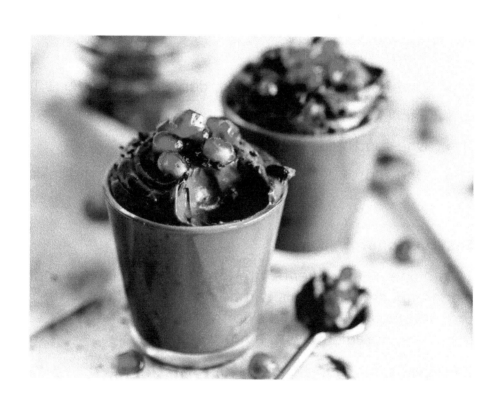

Fresh Strawberry Salad Dressing

Prep Time: 10 minutes

Cook Time: 0 minutes

Serve: 2

Ingredients:

- 1 C – Fresh Ripe Strawberries
- 1 T – Balsamic Vinegar Mosto Cotto 2 T – Lemon Oil
- 1/4 tsp Peppercorns 1 Pinch Sea Salt

Instructions:

1.Put all the ingredients into a food-processor or blender and blend until creamy, then transfer to a serving bowl or pitcher for serving.

Nutrition: Energy (calories): 339 kcal Protein: 0.57 g Fat: 1.83 g Carbohydrates: 82.37 g Calcium, Ca12 mg Magnesium, Mg13 mg Phosphorus, P21 mg

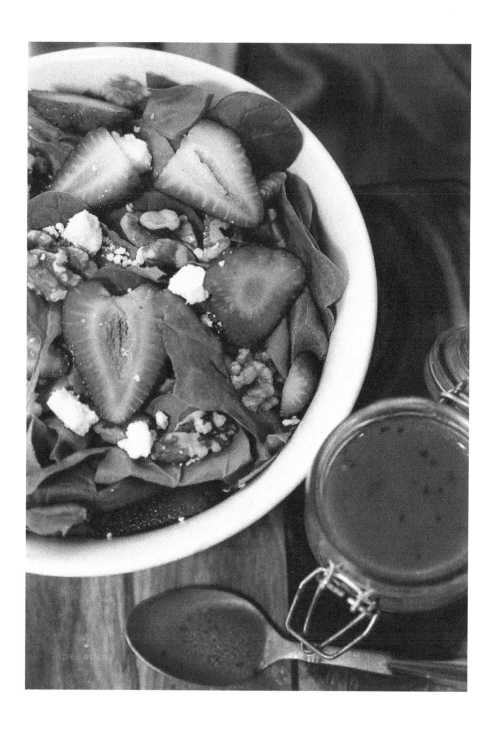

Pumpkin_Balls

Prep Time: 15 minutes

Cook Time: 0 minutes

Serve: 18

Ingredients:

- 1 cup almond butter
- 5 drops liquid stevia
- 2 tbsp coconut flour
- 2 tbsp pumpkin puree
- 1 tsp pumpkin pie spice

Instructions:

1. Mix pumpkin puree in a large bowl and almond butter until well combined.

2. Add liquid stevia, pumpkin pie spice, and coconut flour and mix well.

3. Make little balls from the mixture and place them on a baking tray.

4. Place in the freezer for 1 hour.

Nutrition: Calories: 96 Fat: 8 g Carbs: 4 g Sugar: 1 g Protein: 2 g Cholesterol: 0 mg

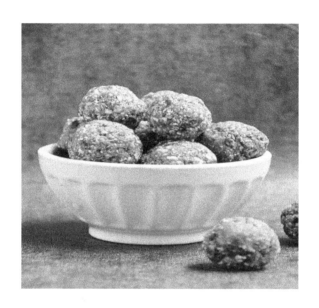

Smooth Peanut Butter Cream

Prep Time: 10 minutes

Cook Time: 0 minutes

Serve: 8

Ingredients:

- 1/4 cup peanut butter
- 4 overripe bananas, chopped
- 1/3 cup cocoa powder
- 1/4 tsp vanilla extract
- 1/8 tsp salt

Instructions:

1. In the blender, add all the listed ingredients and blend until smooth.

Nutrition: Calories: 101 Fat: 5 g Carbs: 14 g Sugar: 7 g Protein: 3 g Cholesterol: 0 mg

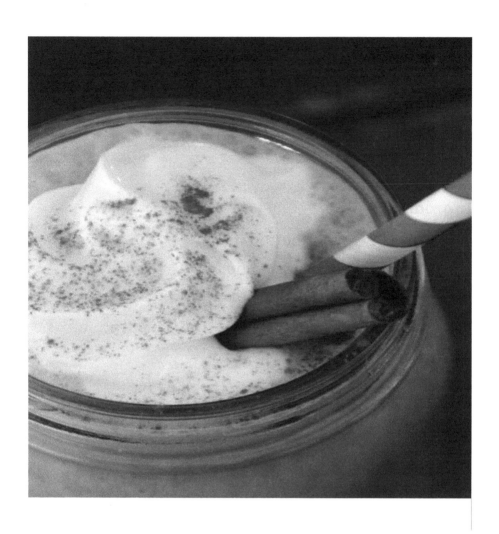

Vanilla Avocado Popsicles

Prep Time: 20 minutes

Cook Time: 0 minutes

Serve: 6

Ingredients:

- 2 avocadoes
- 1 tsp vanilla
- 1 cup almond milk
- 1 tsp liquid stevia
- 1/2 cup unsweetened cocoa powder

Instructions:

1. In the blender, add all the listed ingredients and blend smoothly.

2. Pour blended mixture into the Popsicle molds and place in the freezer until set.

Nutrition: Calories: 130 Fat: 12 g Carbs: 7 g Sugar: 1 g Protein: 3 g Cholesterol: 0 mg

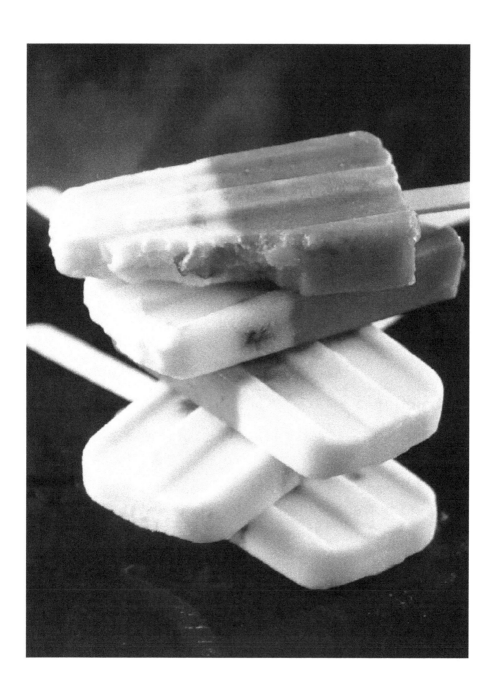

Chocolate Popsicle

Prep Time: 20 minutes

Cook Time: 10 minutes

Serve: 6

Ingredients:

- 4 oz unsweetened chocolate, chopped
- 6 drops liquid stevia
- 1 1/2 cups heavy cream

Instructions:

1. Add heavy cream into the microwave-safe bowl and microwave until it just begins the boiling.

2. Add chocolate into the heavy cream and set aside for 5 minutes.

3. Add liquid stevia into the heavy cream mixture and stir until chocolate is melted.

4. Pour mixture into the Popsicle molds and place in freezer for 4 hours or until set.

Nutrition: Calories: 198 Fat: 21 g Carbs: 6 g Sugar: 0.2 g Protein: 3 g Cholesterol: 41 mg

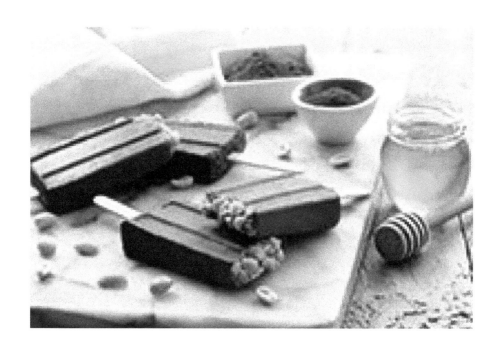

Raspberry Ice Cream

Prep Time: 10 minutes

Cook Time: 0 minutes

Serve: 2

Ingredients:

- 1 cup frozen raspberries
- 1/2 cup heavy cream
- 1/8 tsp stevia powder

Instructions:

1. Blend all the specified ingredients in a blender until smooth.

Nutrition: Calories: 144 Fat: 11 g Carbs: 10 g Sugar: 4 g Protein: 2 g Cholesterol: 41 mg

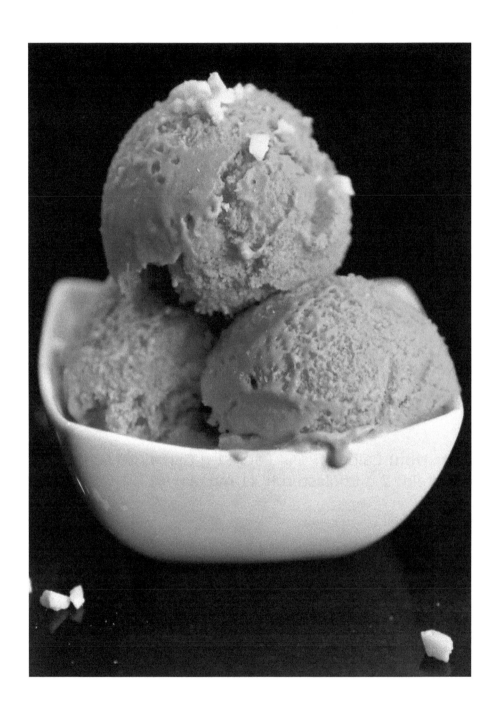

Chocolate Almond Butter Brownie

Prep Time: 10 minutes

Cook Time: 16 minutes

Serve: 4

Ingredients:

- 1 cup bananas, overripe
- 1/2 cup almond butter, melted
- 1 scoop protein powder
- 2 tbsp unsweetened cocoa powder

Instructions:

1. Preheat to 325 F the air fryer. Air fryer baking pan and set aside.

2. Preheat to 325 F the air fryer.

3. In the prepared pan, pour the batter, put it in the air fryer's basket, and cook for 16 minutes.

Nutrition: Calories: 82 Fat: 2 g Carbs: 11 g Sugar: 5 g Protein: 7 g Cholesterol: 16 mg

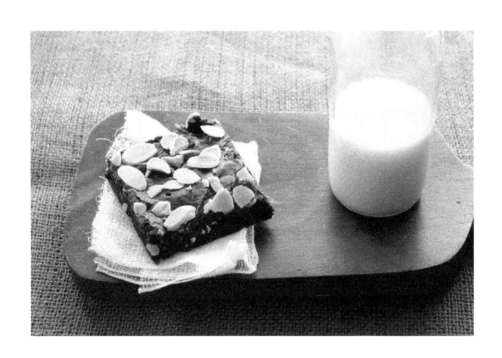

Peanut Butter Fudge

Prep Time: 10 minutes

Cook Time: 10 minutes

Serve: 20

Ingredients:

- 1/4 cup almonds, toasted and chopped
- 12 oz smooth peanut butter
- 15 drops liquid stevia
- 3 tbsp coconut oil
- 4 tbsp coconut cream
- Pinch of salt

Instructions:

1. Line baking tray with parchment paper.

2. In a pan, melt the coconut-oil over low heat. Add peanut butter, coconut cream, stevia, and salt in a saucepan. Stir well.

3. Pour fudge mixture into the prepared baking tray and sprinkle chopped almonds on top.

4. Place the tray in the refrigerator for 1 hour or until set.

Nutrition: Calories: 131 Fat: 12 g Carbs: 4 g Sugar: 2 g Protein: 5 g Cholesterol: 0 mg

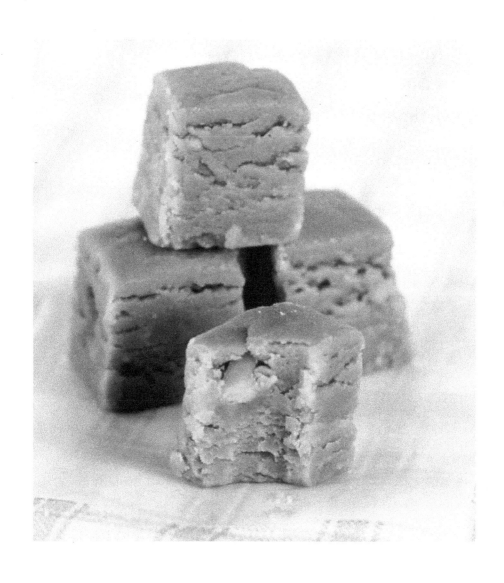

Almond Butter Fudge

Prep Time: 10 minutes

Cook Time: 10 minutes

Serve: 18

Ingredients:

- 3/4 cup creamy almond butter
- 1 1/2 cups unsweetened chocolate chips

Instructions:

1. Line 8*4-inch pan with parchment paper and set aside.

2. Add chocolate chips and almond butter into the double boiler and cook over medium heat until the chocolate-butter mixture is melted. Stir well.

3. place the mixture into the prepared pan and place it in the freezer until set.

Nutrition: Calories: 197 Fat: 16 g Carbs: 7 g Sugar: 1 g Protein: 4 g Cholesterol: 0 mg

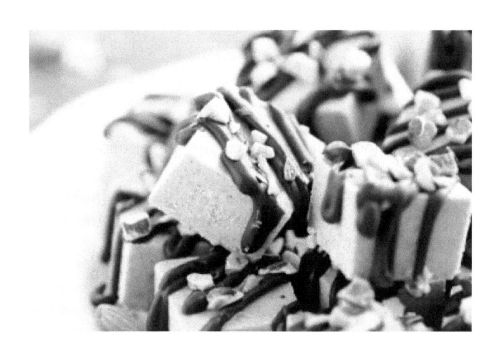

Homemade Coconut Ice Cream

Prep Time: 10 minutes

Cook Time: 95 minutes

Serve: 4

Ingredients:

- 2 cups evaporated low-fat milk
- ⅓ cup low-fat condensed milk
- 1 cup low-fat coconut milk
- 1 cup stevia/xylitol/bacon syrup
- 2 scoops whey protein concentrate
- 2 tsp. sugar-free coconut extract
- 1 tsp. dried coconut

Instructions:

1. Mix all the ingredients together in a bowl.

2. Heat the mixture over medium heat until it starts to bubble.

3. Remove from the heat and then leave the mixture to cool.

4. Chill mixture for about an hour, then freeze in ice cream maker as outlined by the manufacturer's directions.

Nutrition: Calories: 182, Fat: 2 g, Carbohydrates: 20 g, Protein: 22 g

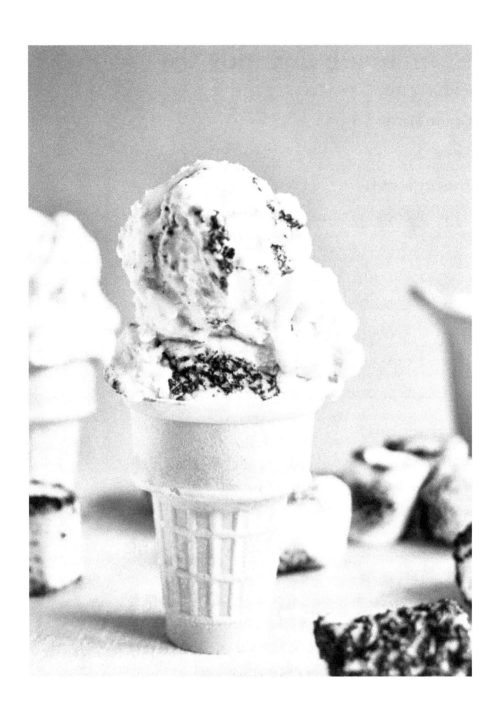

Coconut Panna Cotta

Prep Time: 5 minutes

Cook Time: 20 minutes

Serve: 2

Ingredients:

- 2 cups skimmed milk
- 1/2 cup water
- 1 tsp. sugar-free coconut extract
- 1 envelope powdered grass-fed – organic gelatin – sugar-free
- 2 scoops whey protein isolate
- 4 tbsp. stevia/xylitol/yacon syrup
- ⅓ cup fresh raspberries
- 2 tbsp. fresh mint

Instructions:

1. In a non-stick pan, pour the milk, stevia, water, and coconut Extract.

2. Bring to a boil.

3. Slowly add the gelatin and stir well until the mixtures start to thicken.

4. When ready, divide the mix among the small silicon cups.

5. Refrigerate overnight to relax and hang up.

6. Remove through the fridge and thoroughly turn each cup over ahead of a serving plate.

7. Garnish with raspberries and fresh mint, serve and revel in.

Nutrition: Calories: 130, Fat: 3 g, Carbohydrates: 14 g, Protein: 29 g

Blueberry Lemon Cake

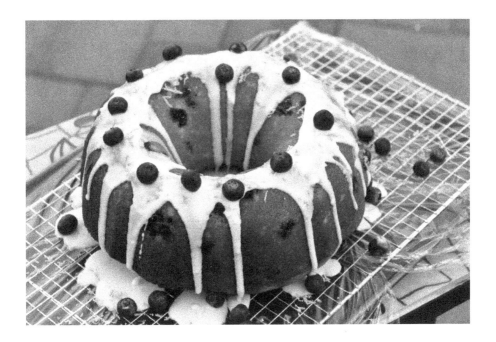

Prep Time: 10 minutes

Cook Time: 40 minutes

Serve: 4

Ingredients:

For the cake:

- 2/3 cup almond flour
- 5 eggs
- ⅓ cup almond milk, unsweetened

- ¼ cup erythritol
- 2 tsp. vanilla extract
- Juice of 2 lemons
- 1 tsp. lemon zest
- ½ tsp. baking soda
- Pinch of salt
- ½ cup fresh blueberries
- 2 tbsp. butter, melted

For the frosting:

- ½ cup heavy cream
- Juice of 1 lemon
- 1/8 cup erythritol

Instructions:

1. Preheat the oven to 35°F

2. In a bowl, add the almond flour, eggs, and almond milk and mix well until smooth.

3. Add the erythritol, a pinch of salt, baking soda, lemon zest, lemon juice, and vanilla extract. Mix and combine well.

4. Fold in the blueberries.

5. Use the butter to grease the pans.

6. Pour the batter into the greased pans.

7. Put on a baking sheet for even baking.

8. Put in the oven to bake until cooked through in the middle and slightly brown on the top, about 35 to 40 minutes.

9. Let cool before removing from the pan.

10. Mix the erythritol, lemon juice, and heavy cream. Mix well.

11. Pour frosting on top.

Nutrition: Calories:274, Fat: 23 g, Carbohydrates: 8 g, Protein: 9 g

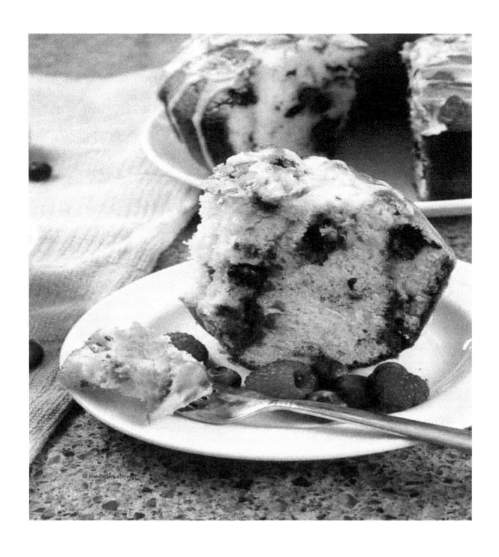

Rich Chocolate Mousse

Prep Time: 10 minutes

Cook Time: 15 minutes

Serve: 3

Ingredients:

- ¼ cup low-fat coconut cream
- 2 cups fat-free Greek-style yogurt, strained
- 4 tsp. powered cocoa, no added sugar
- 2 tbsp. stevia/xylitol/bacon syrup
- 1 tsp. natural vanilla extract

Instructions:

1. Combine all the ingredientsin a medium bowl and mix well.

2. Put individual serving bowls or glasses and refrigerate.

Nutrition: Calories: 269, Fat: 3 g, Carbohydrates: 20 g, Protein: 43 g

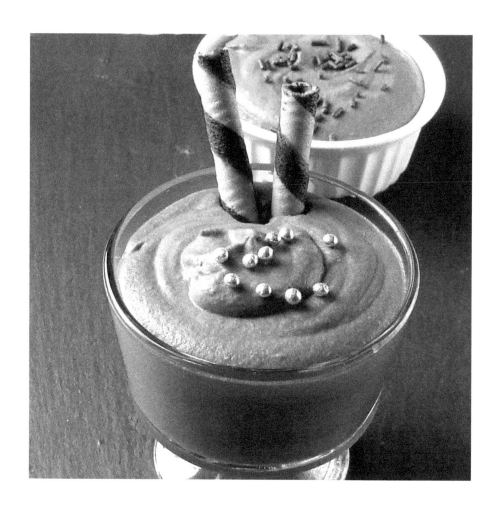

Raspberry Cheesecake

Prep Time: 10 minutes

Cook Time: 25 minutes

Serve: 6

Ingredients:

- 2/3 cup coconut oil, melted
- ½ cup cream cheese
- 6 eggs
- 3 tbsp. granulated sweetener
- 1 tsp. vanilla extract
- ½ tsp. baking powder
- ¾ cup raspberries

Instructions:

1. In a bowl, beat together the coconut oil and cream cheese until smooth.

2. Beat in eggs, then beat in the sweetener, vanilla, and baking powder until smooth.

3. Pour the batter into a pan and finally smooth the top. Scatter the raspberries on top.

4. Bake for 25/30 minutes or until the center is firm.

Nutrition: Calories: 176, Fat: 18 g, Carbohydrates: 3 g, Protein: 6 g

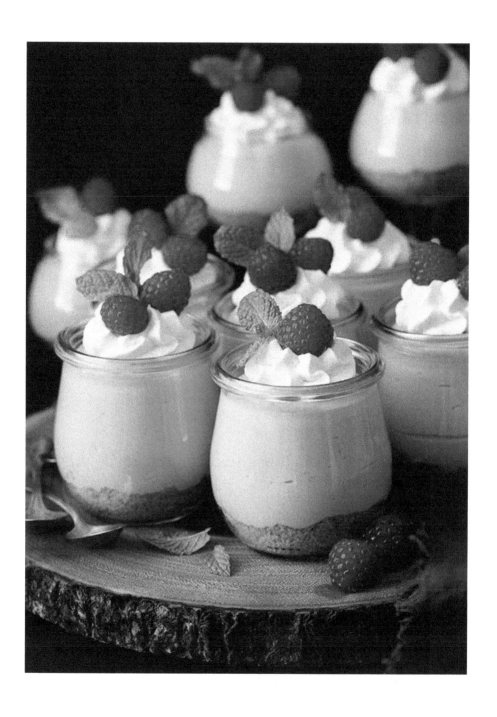

Peanut Butter Brownie Ice Cream Sandwiches

Prep Time: 2 minutes

Cook Time: 2 minutes

Serve: 2

Ingredients:

- 1 packet Medifast Brownie Mix
- 3 tablespoons water
- 1 Peanut Butter Crunch Bar or any bar of your choice
- 2 tablespoons Peanut Butter Powder
- 1 tablespoon water
- 2 tablespoons cool whip

Instructions:

1. Melt the Brownie Mix with water.

2. Add in the Peanut Butter Crunch until a dough is formed.

3. Spoon 4 dough balls on a plate and flatten using the palm of your hands.

4. Make sure that the dough is 1/4 inch thick.

5. Place in a microwave oven and cook for 2 minutes.

6. Meanwhile, mix the Peanut Butter Powder and water to form a paste.

7. Add cool whip. Leave to cool in the fridge for minimun 1 hour.

8. Take the cookies out from the microwave oven and allow it to cool.

9. Once cooled, spoon the peanut butter ice cream in between two cookies.

Nutrition: Calories per serving: 410 Cal, Protein: 8.3 g, Carbohydrates: 57.6 g, Fat: 13.2 g, Sugar: 5.3g

Chocolate Frosty

Prep Time: 20 minutes

Cook Time: 0 minutes

Serve: 4

Ingredients:

- 2 tbsp unsweetened cocoa powder
- 1 cup heavy whipping cream
- 1 tbsp almond butter
- 5 drops liquid stevia
- 1 tsp vanilla

Instructions:

1. Add cream into the medium bowl and beat using the hand mixer for 5 minutes.

2. Add remaining ingredients and blend until thick cream forms.

3. Pour in serving bowls and place them in the freezer for 30 minutes.

Nutrition: Calories: 137 Fat: 13 g Carbs: 3 g Sugar: 0.5 g Protein: 2 g, Cholesterol: 41 mg

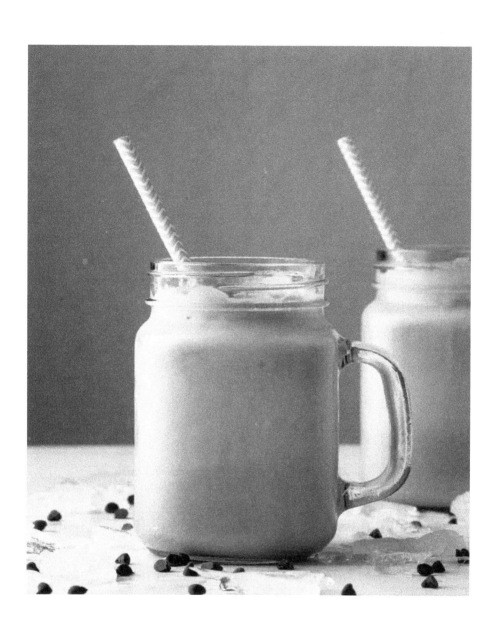

Tiramisu Milkshake

Cook Time: 5 minutes

Serve: 1

Ingredients:

- 1 sachet Frosty Coffee Soft Serve Treat ½ cup ice
- 6 ounces plain low-fat Greek yogurt
- ½ cup almond milk
- 2 tablespoons sugar-free chocolate
- 2 tablespoons whipped topping

Instructions:

1.Place all ingredients, except the whipped, in a blender.

2.Pulse until smooth.

3.Pour in glass and top with whipped topping.

Nutrition: Calories per serving: 239; Protein: 23.7g; Carbs: 64.2g; Fat: 22.8g Sugar: 15.2g

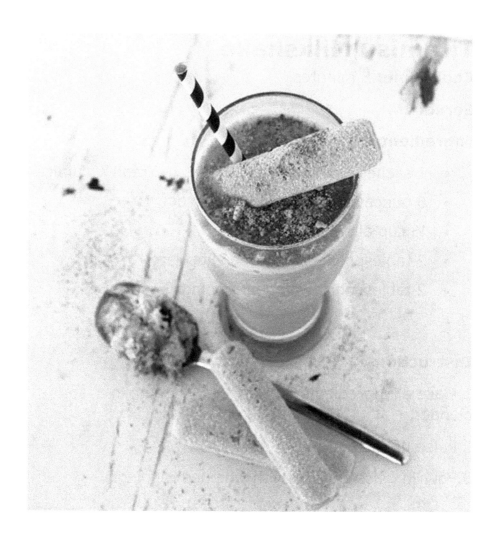

Weight Watchers Macaroni Salad Recipe with Tuna

Prep Time: 15 minutes

Cook Time: 10 minutes

Ingredients:

- 1/2 Cup of Mayonnaise Medium
- 1 tbsp of Red Vinegar
- 1 Tbsp Dijon Mustard
- 1/2 Tbsps Ground Garlic
- 1 Cup of Chopped Celery
- 1/3 Red Onion Cup, Chopped
- 2 Tbsps of Chopped Fresh Parsley
- Salt & Pepper
- 3 Tuna Ounces, In Water
- Macaroni Whole Wheat Elbow (8 Ounces)

Instructions:

1. We must cook the macaroni in salted water first. In order to get the exact times and water measurements, use the kit. Drain the pasta and, after it is cooked, set it aside in a wide tub.

2. When the pasta cooks, the mayonnaise, vinegar, mustard, and garlic powder blend together.

3. Add the mixture of mayonnaise to the cooked pasta, and stir until well mixed.

4. The salmon, celery, cabbage, and parsley are rolled in. Season with salt and pepper to taste.

5. Depending on your tastes, you can serve the dish warm or cold.

Big Mac Salad

Prep Time: 10 minutes

Cook Time: 10 minutes

Ingredients:

Salad Ingredients

- 1 pound lean ground beef
- 1 tsp of Worcestershire sauce
- 1/2 tsp of onion salt
- 1 tsp of minced garlic
- 1 large head romaine, chopped
- 1 large diced tomato
- 1/2 diced small red or white onion
- 1 cup of light cheddar cheese
- 12 diced dill pickles

Dressing Ingredients

- 2 Tbsp of Light Mayo Best Foods or Light Kraft Mayo
- 2 tbsp of nonfat Greek
- 2 tbsp of Ketchup Heinz
- 1/2 tbsp of water
- 1 tbsp of minced white onion
- 1 tsp of sugar
- 1 tsp of sweet pickle relish
- 1 tsp of white vinegar

- dash of salt

Instructions:

1. Spray with non-stick cooking spray on a large skillet. Add the lean ground beef and onion salt and cook, occasionally stirring, for around 5-7 minutes. Using a fork to make the meat crumble.

2. Add sauce from Worcestershire and garlic mined. Stir before the garlic is added. Cook meat until it isn't pink anymore. Take off the heat to cool it down.

3. Measure out 4 ounces of ground beef using a food scale and split equally between the salads. Divide the romaine into four servings, the tomatoes equally.

4. Place 4 ounces of meat on top of lettuce, 1/4 cup cheese, add tomatoes, 2 cups of dressing, and top with diced pickles.

Dressing Ingredients:

1.Whisk or mix light mayonnaise, white vinegar, plain fat or Greek yogurt, sugar ketchup, salt, water, sweet pickle relish, minced white onion, and sugar in a small bowl or in a food processor. Pour into an airtight jar. Place dressing in the refrigerator for a minimum of 30 minutes

Loaded Caesar Salad with Crunchy Chickpeas

Prep Time: 5 minutes

Cook Time: 20 minutes

Serve: 6

Ingredients:

For the chickpeas

- 2 (15-ounce) cans chickpeas, drained and rinsed
- 2 tablespoons extra-virgin olive oil
- 1 teaspoon kosher salt
- 1 teaspoon garlic powder
- 1 teaspoon onion powder
- 1 teaspoon dried oregano

For the dressing

- ½ cup mayonnaise
- 2 tablespoons grated Parmesan cheese
- 2 tablespoons freshly squeezed lemon juice
- 1 clove garlic, peeled and smashed
- 1 teaspoon Dijon mustard
- ½ tablespoon Worcestershire sauce
- ½ tablespoon anchovy paste

For the salad

- 3 heads romaine lettuce, cut into bite-size pieces

Instructions:

To make the chickpeas:

1. Preheat the oven to 450°F. Line a baking sheet with parchment paper.

2. Add the chickpeas, oil, salt, garlic powder, onion powder, and oregano in a small container. Scatter the coated chickpeas on the prepared baking sheet.

3. Roast for about 20 minutes, tossing occasionally, until the chickpeas are golden and have a bit of crunch.

To make the dressing:

1. In a small bowl, whisk the mayonnaise, Parmesan, lemon juice, garlic, mustard, Worcestershire sauce, and anchovy paste until combined.

To make the salad:

1. In a large container combine the lettuce and dressing. Toss to coat. Top with the roasted chickpeas and serve.

Cooking Tip: Don't wash out that bowl you used for the chickpeas — the remaining oil adds a great punch of flavor to blanched green beans or another simply cooked vegetable.

Nutrition: Calories: 367, Total fat: 22 g, Total carbs: 35 g, Cholesterol: 9 mg, Fiber: 13 g, Protein: 12 g, Sodium: 407 mg

Shrimp Cobb Salad

Prep Time: 25 minutes

Cook Time: 10 minutes

Serve: 2

Ingredients:

- 4 slices center-cut bacon
- 1 lb. large shrimp, peeled and deveined
- 1/2 teaspoon ground paprika
- 1/4 teaspoon ground black pepper
- 1/4 teaspoon salt, divided
- 2 1/2 tablespoons fresh lemon juice
- 1 1/2 tablespoons extra-virgin olive oil
- 1/2 teaspoon whole grain Dijon mustard
- 1 (10 oz.) package romaine lettuce hearts, chopped
- 2 cups cherry tomatoes, quartered
- 1 ripe avocado, cut into wedges
- 1 cup shredded carrots

Instructions:

1. Cook the bacon for 4 minutes on each side in a large skillet over medium heat till crispy.

2. Take away from the skillet and place on paper towels; let cool for 5 minutes. Break the bacon into bits. Throw out most of the bacon fat, leaving behind only 1 tablespoon in the skillet.

3. Bring the skillet back to medium-high heat. Add black pepper and paprika to the shrimp for seasoning.

4. Cook the shrimp around 2 minutes each side until it is opaque.

5. Sprinkle with 1/8 teaspoon of salt for seasoning.

6. Combine the remaining 1/8 teaspoon of salt, mustard, olive oil and lemon juice together in a small bowl. Stir in the romaine hearts.

7. On each serving plate, place on 1 and 1/2 cups of romaine lettuce. Add on top the same amounts of avocado, carrots, tomatoes, shrimp and bacon.

Nutrition: Calories: 528, Total Carbohydrate: 22.7 g, Cholesterol: 365 mg, Total Fat: 28.7 g, Protein: 48.9 g, Sodium: 1166 mg

Fruit Salad

Prep Time: 15 minutes

Serve: 4

Ingredients:

For Salad

- 4 cups fresh baby arugula
- 1 cup fresh strawberries, hulled and sliced
- 2 oranges, peeled and segmented

For Dressing

- 2 tablespoons fresh lemon juice
- 2-3 drops liquid stevia
- 2 teaspoons extra-virgin olive oil
- Salt and ground black pepper, as required

Instructions:

1.For Salad: in a salad bowl, place all ingredients and mix.

2.For Dressing: place all ingredients in another bowl and beat until well combined.

3.Place dressing on top of salad and toss to coat well.

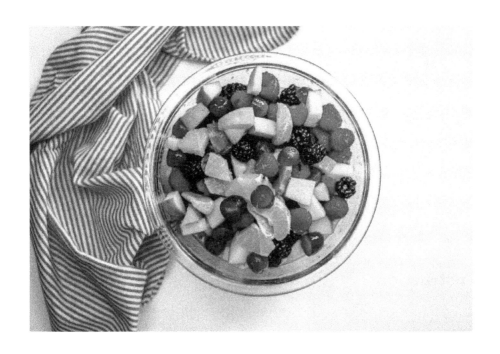

Strawberry, Orange & Rocket Salad

Prep Time: 15 minutes

Serve: 4

Ingredients:

For Salad:

- 6 cups fresh rocket
- 1½ cups fresh strawberries, hulled and sliced 2 oranges, peeled and segmented

For Dressing:

- 2 tablespoons fresh lemon juice
- 1 tablespoon raw honey
- 2 teaspoons extra-virgin olive oil
- 1 teaspoon Dijon mustard
- Salt and ground black pepper, as required

Instructions:

1. For Salad: in a salad bowl, place all ingredients and mix.

2. For Dressing: place all ingredients in another bowl and beat until well combined.

3. Place dressing on top of salad and toss to coat well.

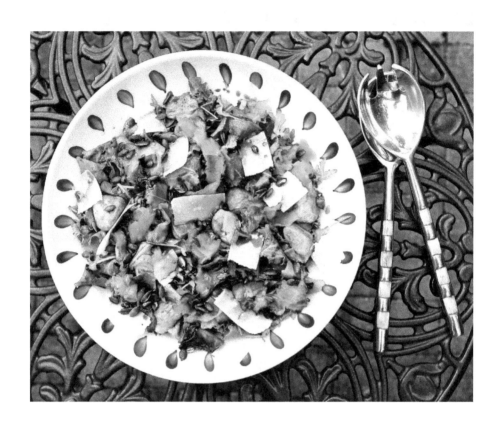

Strawberry & Asparagus Salad

Prep Time: 15 minutes

Cook Time: 5 minutes

Serve: 8

Ingredients:

- 2 pounds fresh asparagus, trimmed and sliced
- 3 cups fresh strawberries, hulled and sliced
- ¼ cup extra-virgin olive oil
- ¼ cup balsamic vinegar
- 2 tablespoons maple syrup
- Salt and ground black pepper, as required

Instructions:

1.In a pan of water, add the asparagus over medium-high heat and bring to a boil.

2.Boil the asparagus for about 2-3 minutes or until al dente.

3.Drain the asparagus and immediately transfer into a bowl of ice water to cool completely.

4.With paper towels, drain the asparagus and pat dry.

5.In a big bowl, add the asparagus and strawberries and mix.

6.In a little bowl, add the olive oil, vinegar, honey, salt and black pepper and beat until well blended.

7. Place the dressing over the asparagus strawberry mixture and gently toss to coat.

8. Refrigerate for about 1 hour before serving.

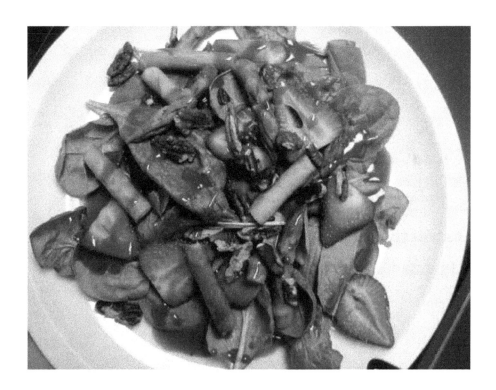

CPSIA information can be obtained
at www.ICGtesting.com
Printed in the USA
BVHW060006310321
603712BV00005B/536

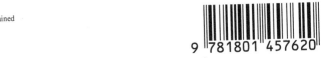